Ketogenic Diet for Beginners:

65 Keto Diet Recipes to Achieve Weight Loss, Ease Type 2 Diabetes, Epilepsy and Prevent Yourself From Cancer

Robin Sandiano

Table of Contents

and is only allowed with express written consent from the Publisher. All additional right reserved.

The information in the following pages is broadly considered to be a truthful and accurate account of facts and as such any inattention, use or misuse of the information in question by the reader will render any resulting actions solely under their purview. There are no scenarios in which the publisher or the original author of this work can be in any fashion deemed liable for any hardship or damages that may befall them after undertaking information described herein.

Additionally, the information in the following pages is intended only for informational purposes and should thus be thought of as universal. As befitting its nature, it is presented without assurance regarding its prolonged validity or interim quality. Trademarks that are mentioned are done without written consent and can in no way be considered an endorsement from the trademark holder.

Introduction

Thank you for downloading *65 Keto Diet Recipes to Achieve Weight Loss, ease Type 2 Diabetes, Epilepsy and Prevent Yourself From Cancer.* Congratulations for taking the initiative to take control of your health.

Some cases of epilepsy are caused by birth defects, brain tumors, stroke, or brain injury, but most cases of epilepsy have unknown etiologies.

Epileptics can be fine one minute and vigorously shaking the next minute and without warning. If these episodes occur at the wrong minute, they can cause physical injuries to the epileptic and sometimes to other people.

Similarly Obesity, Diabetes and Cancer can be caused due to several reasons like Food habits, Unbalanced diet, Heredity etc.

Modern drugs are able to help about 60 to 70% of these sufferers. The other 30 to 40% have Neuro stimulation, surgery, or a Ketogenic diet as options to control the seizures.

While the first version of the ketogenic diet was similar to the Atkins diet, today, there are three main versions of this century-old diet to choose from. Two of the three diets allow some carbohydrate intake, which contributes to a person having the energy to exercise and allows for metabolism of the food.

Reading through the 65 delicious and easy recipes in this book is a great way to get started on the road to better health. You'll likely get excited about several of them and realize that you won't feel as deprived or as chained to the kitchen as you thought you were going to feel.

There are plenty of books on this subject on the market. Thank you again for choosing this one! Every effort was made to ensure it is full of as much useful information as possible. Please enjoy!

Chapter 1: What is the Ketogenic Diet?

The large number of low-carbohydrates on the market today can all trace their efficacy back to the fact that the human body can naturally burn fat for energy. The ketogenic diet consists of a high amount of fat, an adequate amount of protein, and a low amount of carbohydrates.

How it works: The human body can naturally burn fat for energy, the trouble is that most people rarely give it the chance to do so thanks to the high amount of carbohydrates found in their diet. Carbohydrates require less work on the body's part to transform into energy so they will always be consumed first, leaving little need to go after stored fats.

However, you can force your body into a state of ketosis by simply cutting out the amount of glucose available to it for a prolonged period of time until your reserves run dry. After this occurs you will notice an increase in healthy weight loss without having to do anything more than keeping your carb intake level in check.

To understand why this is the case, it is important to consider the average Western diet which typically contains high amounts of carbs, some protein and little healthy fat. Without the fat, it needs to burn energy, the body turns to carbohydrates which are then transformed into glucose which can be used for fuel. The cells in the body then use this glucose to form the molecule ATP which gives the body its energy.

As a result of this process, insulin is also created which has a variety of effects on the body. It helps to get glucose into the bloodstream when it exists in moderation but any leftovers are then turned into fat for use at a later date. As more and more carbs are constantly being introduced to the system, this fat is never used and it builds up and causes weight gain instead.

Once you cut out all the extra carbs, your body enters the ketogenic state and starts the process known as lipolysis which breaks down stored fats into the molecules fatty acid and glycerol which are then utilized by the liver to create energy by generating what are known as Ketones. Ketones then take the place of glucose in most instances where it would be used for energy. When it can't be used as an alternative, the body turns glycerol into glucose and uses it for things like regulating brain functions.

The original diet: This style requires a four-to-one ratio of combined carbohydrates and proteins to fat. As such, you will want to start by cutting out foods that are high in carbohydrates which means no grains, bread, pasta, sugar, and the starchy fruits and vegetables while eating a lot of high-fat foods like butter, cream, and nuts. It gives the body just enough protein to perform its functions of repair and body growth while also providing enough calories for proper weight.

It is the medium-chain triglycerides (MCTs) that are more ketogenic than the common long-chain triglycerides (LCTs), and the original ketogenic diet includes MCTs.

A variant ketogenic diet: A variant of the original diet, which also includes the MCTs, is a diet that replaces much of required fat with a form of coconut oil that is rich in MCTs and gives the dieter half of his calories. Since less fat is needed on this variant form of the diet, more carbs and proteins can be eaten, which widens the variety of food that can be eaten.

Caution: It should be noted that reducing intake of fluids while on one of these diets results in constipation in about 30% of people who restrict fluids. Kidney stones sometimes form as a result, so restriction of fluids is therefore not advised.

Benefits of the Ketogenic Diet

While literally helping to melt the fat off of your body is certainly a great benefit, the keto diet also offers numerous other benefits including literally helping to save your life. It is important to keep in mind that these benefits are only going to accrue while you are in a state of ketosis and the longer that state persists, the more dramatic the results will be.

Reduction of appetite: Besides reducing any fat that might be hanging around, being in a state of ketosis actually reduces feelings of hunger overall which makes it less likely that you will feel the need to continue eating once you start to feel full, thus helping you remain trim without needing to worry about counting calories.

Combats cancers: Many forms of cancer cells feed on excess glucose in the body which means that remaining in a state of ketosis will actually starve these cells, ensuring that they grow much more slowly than they otherwise would. These cancer cells typically have a much greater number of insulin receptor sites when compared to regular cells to help them consume as much glucose as possible. One type of cancer treatment, known as insulin potentiation, takes advantage of this fact and uses ketosis as a means of getting these cells to respond to lower levels of chemotherapy than would otherwise be required. Additionally, these cells have defective mitochondria which leads to the creation of reactive oxygen species, while glucose keeps this process in check, without it these reactive oxygen species actually kill the cancer cells.

Eases type 2 diabetes effects: Ketosis is also a useful means of those with type 2 diabetes to reduce their glucose levels which can also reduce their reliance on external insulin. Those with the disease are typically pushed towards a low carb diet anyway due to the fact that they become sugar when converted to energy. Switching to foods that focus on fats can thus cause a reduction in blood sugar.

Treats epilepsy: It is also known to help combat epilepsy and nearly half of the children and young people who have been on the ketogenic diet experienced far fewer epileptic seizures. In fact, the number of seizures dropped by more than half and the benefits lasted after they were off of the diet. This diet has shown evidence that it can reduce the episodes of epileptic seizures in adults too when a less strict form of the diet is used. The results of current research studies suggest that the ketogenic diet protects neurons and modifies diseases for many adults who have neurodegenerative disorders. Still, the use of the diet to treat any form of epilepsy other than pediatric epilepsy is considered to still be in the research stage.

Other benefits of the ketogenic diet are increased energy, improved performance, mental clarity, improved cognitive function, better digestion, and a slowdown of the aging process.

Types of Ketogenic Diet

There are three main forms of the ketogenic diet today. Each one caters to particular circumstances that people have. The main issue with both the Atkins and the traditional (Standard) ketogenic diet is that the strict reduction in carbohydrates greatly reduces a person's energy level, making an intense workout in a gym hard to do. The variations that now exist tweak keto so that some carbohydrates can regularly be eaten, which attracts many people back to the ketogenic diet.

Standard Ketogenic Diet (SKD) – This is the form of the diet that continually calls for a high amount of fats, a low amount of carbs, and a moderate amount of protein every day. It is similar to the Atkins diet and is the form of the diet most people are familiar with. Its purpose is to establish ketosis, which reduces the frequency of epileptic seizures in addition to enabling weight loss.

Milk, fruit, and starches are not allowed on this diet, and the dieter eats a lot of butter, oils, cheese, and fatty cuts of meat. This diet is followed for seven days a week without exception.

The person can work out any time during the diet, but the person would not have much energy because they wouldn't have eaten much in the way of carbohydrates. Under 30 grams of carbs are allowed on this diet. Many of the recipes in this book include food with up to 30 grams of carbohydrates.

Therefore, the SKD is not recommended for people who work out regularly or for people who would not be self-disciplined enough to follow a strict diet.

This diet is recommended for sedentary people, for people who are extremely obese, and for anybody who would have a hard time exercising. This diet controls the urges for carbohydrates, regulates hunger, and effectively starts the process of fat loss without exercise.

A low number of calories for an extended period can cause the metabolism to slow down, preventing the dieter from losing more weight. Without an occasional high-carb day, the fat loss hormones of Leptin and Ghrelin would not be reset, so a person should not stay on this diet indefinitely.

After the weight has been lost and the person is able to exercise, then he or she can switch to one of the other two forms of the ketogenic diet which allow more carbohydrates, which enables more activity and resets the fat loss hormones.

Targeted Ketogenic Diet (TKD) – This form of the diet allows the person to consume between 25 and 50 grams of carbs whenever the person works out. The carbs are to be just enough to sustain the person during the workout without affecting the ketosis.

This is actually an SKD with the added carbs and workout around three times per week, usually every other day. This diet is good for the person who is disciplined enough to exercise three times per week.

Cyclical Ketogenic Diet (CKD) – This form of the diet calls for the strict version of the diet for five days of the week and binging on carbs on the other two days.

Whether or not the dieter exercises, this form of the diet is meant to make the dieter stick to the diet because it is easier to live with than one that never allows them to have many carbs. People on this diet usually utilize the weekends for their binge days, going out to dinner, drinking beer, etc., and then get back to the business of dieting during the work week.

How this Book Can Help?

The ketogenic diet does not have to consist of boring or complicated recipes. They can be very simple dishes. Delicious and often very simple recipes are what make this ketogenic cookbook different from other ketogenic cookbooks. There are some longer recipes included in here also, however, for variety.

You now know that you have some dietary options that allow for the consumption of carbohydrates, which would give you the energy to work out at the gym or would merely help you to stay on a diet.

Some recipes include more carbohydrates than other recipes do. These higher-carbohydrate recipes accommodate people who need extra energy to exercise and people who are on their weekend binge time, but not wanting to go too far off of the plan.

Note: Most of the recipes include the numbers for their calories, carbohydrates, fats, and so on, but others do not include them. The ones that do not have that information tend to be recipes for foods that have high fat-to-carb ratios, which is more suitable for the standard ketogenic diet.

Chapter 2: Breakfast Recipes

Bacon and Eggs

Fat: 20 g | Protein: 12 g | Calories:250 | Fiber:1 g | Carbs: 3 g |

This recipe needs 12 minutes to cook and will make 1 serving.

What to Use

- Bacon (3 strips)
- Eggs (3)
- Sea salt (to taste)
- Garlic powder (to taste)
- Onion powder (to taste)

What to Do

- Fry the bacon. Take the cooked bacon out of the pan and put it on a plate covered with paper towel.
- Fry the eggs in the bacon fat.
- Season the eggs while frying.

Bacon, Eggs and Veggie Breakfast

Fat: 16 g | Protein: 10 g | Calories:180 | Fiber:2 g | Carbs: 5 g |

This recipe needs 10 minutes to prepare, 22 minutes to cook, and will make 2   servings.

What to Use

- Eggs (4 large)
- Broccoli (.5 cups, hashed)
- Celery (.5 cups)
- Onion (.5 of white onion, hashed)
- Carrot (1, shredded)
- Cheese (.5 cup, shredded)
- Butter (1 tablespoon)
- Bacon (8 slices)

What to Do

- Shred the carrot and the cheese. Set aside.
- Chop the broccoli, celery and the half of an onion. Set aside.
- Cut the bacon across the grain into several pieces.

- Add the butter to the frying pan before placing it on a burner turned to a medium heat.
- Stirring frequently, sauté the carrot and broccoli along with the celery until the bacon reaches your desired level of crispness or the vegetables start to caramelize.
- Spread everything out evenly on the bottom of the frying pan except for in four corners of the pan.
- Break an egg into each cleared corner of the frying pan. Cover if you want the yolks cooked. Leave uncovered if you don't. Turn egg over once.
- When the eggs are almost cooked through, spread the veggies with the cheese. Turn off the heat and let the cheese melt.

Broccoli and Cheese Omelet

*Fat: 8g | Protein: 20g | Calories:183 | Fiber:2g | Carbs: 6g
|*

This recipe needs 15 minutes to prepare 5 minutes to cook
and will make 1 serving.

What to Use

- Salt (as desired)
- Pepper (as desired)
- Egg (1)
- Egg whites (2)
- Skim milk (1 T)
- Broccoli (.5 cup, cooked)
- Swiss cheese (1 slice)

What to Do

- Chop and cook the broccoli.
- Separate the yolk from two of the eggs. Whisk the
  eggs along with the egg whites before mixing in the
  milk, salt, and pepper and stir together.
- Use a cooking oil spray on a frying pan before placing
  it on a burner turned to a medium heat.

- Add in the seasoned egg and milk mixture. Reduce the heat.
- Put the slice of cheese in the middle of the eggs.
- Put the broccoli on top of the cheese.
- Flip the sides into the middle when the eggs are set to create an omelet.

Caramelized Onion, Red Pepper, and Zucchini Frittata

Calories: 157 | Fat: 8.3g | Protein: 14.6g | Carbs: 5.9g | Fiber: 2.6g

This recipe needs 10 minutes preparation, 28 minutes cooking time, and will serve 4.

What to Use

- Onion (1 white, thinly sliced rings)
- Red pepper (1 medium, diced)
- Zucchini (1.5 cups, diced into matchsticks)
- Eggs (4 large)
- Egg whites (4 large egg whites)
- Parmesan cheese (.25 cup, grated)
- Olive oil (as needed)
- Pepper (as desired)
- Salt (as desired)

What to Do

- Chop up the onion, red pepper and zucchini.
- Heat up the oil in the skillet.
- Fry up the onion about 10 minutes.

- Sprinkle peppers and cook about 5 more minutes.
- Add zucchini peppers, salt, and pepper and cook about 3 more minutes.
- Mix together the eggs along with the egg whites and seasonings in a mixing bowl.
- Pour the eggs into the skillet, distributed evenly over the vegetables.
- Cook about 2 minutes and add the pan into the oven.
- Bake approximately 12 minutes.

Coconut Oil-Fried Eggs and Veggies

Calories: 234 | Fat: 11g | Protein: 13g | Carbs: 4.8g | Fiber: 1.3g

This recipe needs 10 minutes to cook and will make 2 servings.

What to Use

- Eggs (3 – 4)
- Coconut oil (as needed)
- Mixed frozen vegetable (small bag, frozen)
- Salt (as desired)
- Pepper (as desired)
- Spinach (to taste)
- Other seasonings (as desired)

What to Do

- Heat up the coconut oil in a frying pan.
- Add veggies. Stir to coat.
- Add eggs.
- Stir fry until cooked.

Egg White Spinach Omelet

Calories: 301g | Fat: 10g | Protein: 15.1g | Carbs: 10g | Fiber: .9g

This recipe needs 8 minutes to prepare, 5 minutes to cook, and will make 2   servings.

What to Use

- Almond milk (30 milliliters)
- Tomato (.5 of tomato)
- Purple onion (1 tabs)
- Egg whites (of 4 – 5 eggs)
- Egg yolks (from 1 egg)
- Spinach (1 handful, shredded)
- Basil (1 pence)
- Olive oil cooking spray
- Garlic (optional)

What to Do

- Chop up the tomato and the onion. Set aside.
- In a separate bowl beat the egg whites, egg yolk and the almond milk.

- Add cooking oil to a frying pan before placing it on a burner turned to a medium heat.
- Sauté the chopped veggies just enough to soften them and pull them from the pan.
- Re-prepare the pan and then add in the beaten eggs and fry them over medium heat unto firm.
- Fold the sautéed veggies into the egg.
- Serve as is or with fresh fibrous or citrus fruit (adds calories the listed amount)

Eggs Benedict with Lazy Hollandaise Sauce

Calories: 568 | Fat: 55.9g | Protein: 15.5g | Carbs: 2.1g | Fiber: 0.5g

This recipe needs 5 minutes to prepare, 5 minutes to cook, and will serve 1.

What to Use

- Butter (2 tablespoons)
- Egg (1)
- Ham (1 slice)
- Lazy Hollandaise Sauce

What to Do

- Heat up butter in a frying pan.
- Cook egg in an egg ring or scramble with a little manipulation, flipping once.
- Fold egg over if not cooked in a ring.
- Cut ham to fit the size of the egg when folded or the size of the egg ring.
- Put ham onto a serving plate. Put the egg on top.
- Top off with hollandaise sauce (see below).

What to Use (to Make the Lazy Hollandaise Sauce)

- Lemon juice (1 tsp)
- Mayonnaise (.25 c)
- Pepper (as desired)

What to Do (to Make Lazy Hollandaise Sauce)

- Blend all ingredients.

Kale, Ricotta Cheese and Squash Omelet

Calories: 87 | Fat: 6.2g | Protein: 5.2g | Carbs: 3g | Fiber: .9g

This recipe needs 8 minutes of preparation time, 11 minutes of cooking time, and will make 1-2 servings.

What to Use

- Eggs (2 large, free-range)
- Kale (1 handful, fresh or frozen kale powder)
- Ricotta cheese (2 tablespoons)
- Butternut squash (150 g, roasted)
- Olive oil (as needed)
- Parmesan cheese (to taste)

What to Do

- Whisk the eggs in a bowl.
- Blend fresh kale in a blender until fine.
- Add the kale and the ricotta cheese to the bowl of whisked eggs.
- Take the skin off of the squash. Mash the squash and add it to the bowl.
- Preheat grill to medium-high.

- Put a little oil in the bottom of a non-stick frying pan and ensure the whole thing is well-coated.
- Place the frying pan on top of a burner set to a medium heat.
- Pour mixture into hot frying pan and spread it out evenly.
- Cook mixture 1 or 2 minutes or until the sides start to get golden in color.
- Put grated parmesan on the omelet. Grill 3 to 5 minutes.
- Add a dash of black pepper and sea salt to taste.

Keto Pancakes

Calories: 327 | Fat: 10.2g | Protein: 5.3g | Carbs: 8.2g | Fiber: 6.7g

This recipe needs 8 minutes of preparation time, 11 minutes of cooking time, and will make 2 servings.

What to Use

- Almond milk (3 tablespoons plus 1 teaspoon)
- Coconut oil (2 T + 1 tsp)
- Coconut flour (2 T)
- Caramel syrup (.5 teaspoon)
- Protein powder (.75 cup)
- Butter (2 cubes, softened but not melted)
- Sugar (.75 cup), or *a sugar substitute*
- Egg yolk (1 large, yolk separated)
- Vanilla essence (.5 teaspoon)
- Salt (per taste)
- Baking powder (1 teaspoon)

What to Do

- Mix the salt, sugar, baking powder and the flour together in a bowl.

- Make a "well" in the middle of the dry mixture. Pour in the almond milk, caramel syrup, vanilla essence, protein powder and the egg yolk.
- Mix the protein powder and liquid ingredients together and then mix that mixture in with the dry ingredients until all ingredients are well blended, but not overly blended, together.
- Add coconut oil to a frying pan before placing it on a burner turned to a medium heat.
- Cook pancakes and serve with butter cubes.

Pumpkin Waffles

Calories: 243 | Fat: 21g | Protein: 9g | Carbs: 3.8g | Fiber: 6.2g

This recipe needs 6 minutes of preparation time, 11 minutes of cooking time, and will make 1 serving.

What to Use

- Flax seed meal (6 – 7 tablespoons)
- Almond meal (8 tablespoons)
- Eggs (2 – 3)
- Coconut milk (6 tablespoons, thick, unsweetened)
- Butter (1.5 tablespoons)
- Pumpkin puree (3 tablespoons, pure)

What to Do

- Measure out and mix all ingredients together, being careful not to make the batter too thick or too runny.
- Heat up the waffle iron.
- Put batter in the iron. Cook. Turn the waffle iron over and cook a little longer.

Raspberry Protein Shake

Calories: 205 | Fat: 7.3g | Protein: 19.8g | Carbs: 2.9g | Fiber: 5.4g

This recipe needs 10 minutes to prepare and will make 1 - 2 servings.

What to Use

- Natural peanut butter (24 grams)
- Almond milk (1 cup)
- Raspberries (77 grams)
- Strawberry protein powder (1 scoop)
- Ground coffee (1 teaspoon, optional)
- Cinnamon (.25 teaspoon)
- Ginger (.25 teaspoon)

What to Do

- Blend the raspberries in the blender. Add the almond milk, then the protein powder, peanut butter, cinnamon and the ginger.
- Add coffee if desired. Blend until smooth.

Roasted Chilli Frittata

Calories: 578 | Fat: 48.3g | Protein: 14.6g | Carbs: 3g | Fiber: 9g

This recipe needs 20 minutes to prepare, 10 minutes to cook, and will make 2   servings.

What to Use

- Grated parmesan cheese (10 grams)
- Chillies (4-8 chillies, a mixture of green)
- Green pepper
- Parsley (6 sprigs, flat-leaf)
- Butter (1 knob)
- Free-range eggs (5 large)
- Goat cheese (100 g)
- Coconut oil (4 T divided)
- Garlic clove (1 hashed)
- Salad greens (as needed)
- Ham, prosciutto, or bacon

What to Do

- Preheat oven on high.
- Prick chillies.

- Blacken chillies over flame. Place them into a medium-sized mixing bowl before covering using plastic wrap and letting them sit for approximately 12 minutes.
- Prepare the chillies for use before tearing them into strips and returning to the bowl.
- Mix the parsley and the 2 T coconut oil into the mixing bowl.
- Add the remaining coconut oil to a skillet before placing it on a burner turned to a medium heat.
- Add the chopped garlic and half of the marinated chillies.
- In a separate bowl, add in the eggs and seasonings and beat well.
- Finely chop most, but not all, of the parsley leaves. Add the chopped parsley to the second bowl.
- Add the results to the skillet. Next, add cheese by crumbling the feta cheese or the goat's cheese into the eggs.
- Fry until the egg starts to set up. Crumble the rest of the cheese into the skillet.
- Bake 5 minutes or until it is twice its size.
- Take out of the oven. Drizzle some of the chili marinade on top.

- Sprinkle with the remaining parsley.
- Serve with ham, prosciutto or bacon.

Spicy Omelet

Calories: 280 | Fat: 17g | Protein: 36g | Carbs: 4g | Fiber: 3.5g

This recipe needs 15 minutes to prepare, 6 minutes to cook, and will make 2   servings.

What to Use

- Shrimp (10 large)
- Spinach (.125 pound)
- Tomatoes (4 grape)
- Eggs (6)
- Coconut oil (1 tablespoon and 1 teaspoon)
- Onion (one)
- Parsley (1 spring)
- Cayenne (.25 teaspoon)
- Salt (as desired)
- Pepper (as desired)

What to Do

- Chop the spinach and half of the onion.
- Slice the tomatoes.

- Add the coconut oil to a frying pan before placing it on a burner turned to a medium heat.
- Add in onion, sliced tomatoes, and any desired seasonings.
- After the onions become clear, add the chopped spinach and cook until all ingredients have shrunk.
- Add the shrimp to the pan.
- Separate the yolks from the eggs and add just the yolks to the pan.
- Cover the pan and briefly let cook. Turn the omelet over to cook on the other side. Total cook time is only 5.
- Top with parsley prior to serving.

Keto Tortillas

Calories: 98 | Fat: 2.1g | Protein: 3.2g | Carbs: 4.1g | Fiber: 1.2g

This recipe needs 2.5 hours to prepare, 12 minutes to cook, and will make 2 – 4 servings.

What to Use

- Flax seed meal (1 cup)
- Husk powder (2 tablespoons)
- Olive oil (2 tablespoons)
- Xanthan gum (.25 tablespoon)
- Curry powder (.5 tablespoon)
- Filtered water (1 cup)
- Coconut water (1 tablespoon)
- Coconut flour (.5 tablespoon)

What to Do

- Put the flax seed meal, Xanthan gum, psyllium husk powder and a dash of curry powder into a bowl. Mix well.

- Mix in the water along with the olive oil. Mix well and then leave uncovered for at least an hour so that the flax would have time to absorb the other ingredients.
- Divide the mixture into five parts. With a Silpat, press each of the portions on your hand.
- Add a dash of coconut oil to each tortilla as you work with them and roll them out as thinly as possible.
- Use a large round object as a guide to cut off excess tortilla dough.
- Over medium heat, heat up a small amount of olive oil.
- Fry a tortilla until brown. Add more oil and repeat for each tortilla.
- Fry up some bacon, mushrooms, or vegetables to serve with the tortillas.

Chapter 3: Lunch Recipes

Asian-Inspired Chicken Wings

Calories: 320 | Fat: 8.3g | Protein: 17.1g | Carbs: 5.6g | Fiber: 2.6g

This recipe needs 15 minutes to prepare, 24 hours to marinate, 1 hour to cook, and will make several servings.

What to Use

- Chicken wings (3 pounds, separated)
- Fennel seed (1 tsp)
- Ginger (.5 tablespoon, fresh, chopped)
- Fish sauce (1 T)
- Coconut aminos (.5 cup), or substitute reduced-sodium tamari soy sauce
- Extra virgin coconut oil (2 T)
- Anise seed (1 tsp.)
- Apple cider vinegar (2 T)
- Sesame oil (2 tablespoons)
- Honey (2 T)
- Garlic cloves (4 hashed)

What to Do

- Pat the chicken dry and place into a large bowl. Alternatively, a large resealable bag would work to marinate the chicken in.
- Add the coconut oil to a saucepan before placing it over a burner set to a high-medium heat.
- Mix in ginger, garlic, anise, and the fennel seed. Stir constantly 2 to 3 minutes.
- Add the coconut aminos, vinegar, honey, and the fish sauce. Boil before letting it simmer for 60 seconds before removing from the burner.
- Pour in the sesame oil before mixing well.
- Add the results to the tops of the chicken wings and ensure they are well-coated. Let cool.
- Cover and let them marinate for 24 hours in the refrigerator, stirring once or twice while marinating. If using a bag, just flip it over.
- Drain off the excess marinade.
- Put them on your grill and cook for about 20 minutes, turning once. Alternatively ensure your oven is heated to 375 degrees Fahrenheit, put on tin foil on a cookie sheet, place wings on cookie sheet and bake for 1 hour.

Bacon, Egg, Avocado and Tomato Salad

Calories: 157 | Fat: 12.2g | Protein: 12.1g | Carbs: 8.6g | Fiber: 9.1g

This recipe needs 20 minutes to prepare and will make 1 serving.

What to Use

- Avocado (1 ripe, chopped)
- Eggs (2 boiled, chopped)
- Tomato (1 medium, chopped)
- Lemon juice (from 1 wedge)
- Salt (as desired)
- Pepper (as desired)
- Bacon (2-4 slices, cooked and crumbled, optional)

What to Do

- Combine all of ingredients together is a salad bowl and mix slightly so egg and avocado are a little mushy.

Bacon-Wrapped Mini Meatloaves

Calories: 350| Fat: 8.9g | Protein: 21.2g | Carbs: 10.8g | Fiber: 4.4g

This recipe needs 20 minutes of preparation, 30 minutes of cooking time, and will serve 4.

What to Use

- Ground beef (1 pound)
- Bacon (.5 pound, cut into small chunks)
- Bacon (8 additional full strips)
- Coconut milk (.25 cup)
- Garlic (2 cloves, minced)
- Chives (.33 cup, fresh, minced)
- Salt (as desired)
- Pepper (as desired)
- Parsley (to taste, fresh, chopped)

What to Do

- Ensure oven is heated to 400 degrees F.
- Combine the coconut milk, ground beef, bacon chunks, chives and the garlic in a large mixing bowl. Mix well. All ingredients should hold together.

- Season with ground black pepper. No salt would be needed.
- Wrap a piece of bacon around the sides of each hole in a mini muffin tin.
- Fill the holes with the beef mixture.
- Bake for 30 minutes.
- Let cool. Remove and serve with fresh parsley on top.

BLT Chicken Salad

Calories: 475 | Fat: 31g | Protein: 42g | Carbs: 7g | Fiber: 2g

This recipe needs 22 minutes to prepare, 30 minutes to cook, and will make 1   serving.

What to Use

- Boneless chicken breast (1, grilled)
- Leaf lettuce (2 cups, chopped)
- Tomato (.5 small)
- Swiss cheese (.5-ounce, julienned)
- Bacon (1-2 strips, crisp and crumbled)
- Egg (.5 hard boiled, sliced in half)
- Ranch dressing (2 tablespoons)
- Black pepper (dash)
- Parsley (pinch, fresh, chopped, optional)
- Sliced cucumber (chopped, optional)
- Chives (chopped, optional)
- Green peppers (slivered, optional)
- Avocado (chopped, optional)
- Sunflower seeds (optional)

What to Do

- Add the chicken to the grill and let it cook until the internal temperature reaches 165 degrees F. Slice it thinly.
- Add the sliced chicken to a large plate covered in lettuce.
- Top the chicken with the remaining ingredients.

Bora Bora Meatballs

Calories: 230 | Fat: 14.5g | Protein: 15.3g | Carbs: 5.1g | Fiber: 1.9g

This recipe needs 8 minutes of preparation time, 11 minutes of cooking time, and will make 42 meatballs.

What to Use

- Ground pork (2 pounds)
- Unsweetened shredded coconut (1.5 cups)
- Salt (as desired)
- Pepper (as desired)
- Cayenne pepper (1.75 teaspoons, ground)
- Jalapeno (2 teaspoons, seeded, minced fine, de-ribbed)
- Crushed pineapple (1 c. DO NOT USE FRESH PINEAPPLE)
- Coconut aminos (2 tablespoons)
- Ginger (1.5 teaspoons, dried)
- Garlic (3 cloves/1 tablespoons, minced)
- Scallions (.25 cup sliced thin)
- Eggs (2 large, beaten lightly)

What to Do

- Ensure oven is heated to 375 degrees F.
- Prepare a baking sheet before covering it with aluminum foil.
- Place a non-stick skillet on top of a burner set to a high-medium heat.
- Place the coconut in the skillet and let it cook about 3 minutes, often stirring until golden brown. Remove the skillet from atop the burner.
- Seasons as needed. Remove the results from the skillet and place it into a bowl.
- Drain the pineapple over something that catches the juice, pressing most of the juice out of it. Save the juice.
- Put the pineapple into a third bowl. Add 1 teaspoon of cayenne and .5 teaspoon of salt. Also add the coconut aminos, ginger, scallions, garlic, eggs, and the jalapeno. Mix well.
- Crumble the pork into the pineapple mixture. Wash your hands and then knead until well mixed.
- Arrange the three bowls (seasoned pork, pineapple juice, and spiced coconut), so they can be easily accessed.

- Measure out 1 T of pork. Roll into a ball, coat using the juice from the pineapple and coat thoroughly using the coconut. Place meatballs .5 inch apart on the baking sheet.
- Place the baking sheet in the oven and let it cook approximately 30 minutes until the meatballs are well-browned.
- Plate with oven-roasted cauliflower rice.

Broccoli Soup

Calories: 207 | Fat: 13g | Protein: 11g | Carbs: 8g | Fiber: 2.3g

This recipe needs 30 minutes to prepare, 40 minutes to cook, and will make several servings.

What to Use

- Butter (1 tablespoon)
- Onion (.5, white)
- Garlic (1 teaspoon, minced)
- Heavy cream (1.75 cups plus 2 tablespoons)
- Broth (.5 cup plus 2 tablespoons)
- Water (.5 cup plus 2 tablespoons)
- Broccoli (1.5 cups)
- Cheddar cheese (8 ounces)
- Salt and pepper (to taste)
- Paprika (.5 teaspoon)
- Xanthan Gum (.25 teaspoon)

What to Do

- Chop up the onion and the broccoli.

- Add the butter to a large pot before placing it on top of a burner set to a medium heat.
- Sauté the onion with the garlic together for about 3 minutes.
- Mix in the water, cream, and the broth. Bring to boil.
- Mix in the broccoli and the spices.
- Leave the pot be for 25 minutes.
- Add the cheese.
- Cool enough to put into the blender without shattering it.
- Add the gum. Blend well.
- Pour into serving bowls. Garnish with more cheddar cheese.

California Grilled Chicken Avocado-Mango Salad

Calories: 258 | Fat: 14.6g | Protein: 22g | Carbs: 12.2g | Fiber: 3.8g

This recipe needs 15 minutes to prepare and will make 4 servings.

What to Use

- Chicken breast (12-ounce breast, grilled, sliced)
- Avocado (1 cup, diced)
- Mango (1 cup, diced from 1.5 mangos)
- Red onion (2 tablespoons)
- Red butter lettuce (6 cups)

What to Do

- Make the vinaigrette (See below) and set aside.
- Fill 4 salad plates with baby greens.
- Toss the onion, mango, avocado, and chicken together.
- Plate the chicken atop the baby greens and top with vinaigrette prior to serving.

*What to Use (to Make **Vinaigrette**)*

- balsamic vinegar (2 tablespoons white)
- Salt (as desired)
- Pepper (as desired)
- Olive oil (2 T)

*What to Do (to Make **Vinaigrette**)*

- Whisk all ingredients together. Set aside.

Chef Salad Ham Cups

Calories: 310 | Fat: 12.9g | Protein: 15.8g | Carbs: 7.2g | Fiber: 1.2g

This recipe needs 10 minutes preparation, 28 minutes cooking time, and will serve 1.

What to Use

- Cheddar cheese (.5 cups shredded)
- Ham (2 thin slices)
- Lettuce (shredded)
- Tomato (chopped)
- Egg (1 hard-boiled, sliced)

What to Do

- Ensure your oven is heated to 350 degrees Fahrenheit.
- Put muffin pan or custard cups on a cookie sheet.
- Put the 2 ham slices on top of an inverted muffin pan or custard cups in an x shape.
- Place the second custard on top of the first one, so the ham won't overcook. You are creating a "bowl" out of the ham.

- Cut off the excess ham. Leave 1.2 inches. The ham will shrink.
- Bake 20 minutes.
- Once it has finished cooking, let it cool for 15 minutes.
- Remove top bowl. Cool. Remove bottom bowl when cool enough.
- Fill ham cup with the lettuce, egg, tomato and the cheese.
- Serve cold.

Chicken Soup

Calories: 280 | Fat: 32g | Protein: 15g | Carbs: 4.2g | Fiber: 8g

This recipe needs 15 minutes to prepare, 20 minutes to cook, and will make 1 serving.

What to Use

- Salt (as desired)
- Pepper (as desired)
- Chicken (6 ounces, shredded)
- Celery stalks (3)
- Olive oil (40 milliliters)
- Cayenne (.5 tsp powdered)
- Bell pepper (1, red)
- Garlic (1 teaspoon, minced)
- Chicken broth (200 milliliters)
- Tomatoes (1 cup, diced)
- Cream cheese (6 ounces)
- Cilantro (2 ounces)
- Cumin (1 tsp)

What to Do

- Dice the celery and the bell pepper.
- Add the olive oil to a skillet before placing the skillet on top of a burner set to a medium heat.
- Add in celery, bell pepper, and the garlic until the celery softens.
- Season as desired.
- Mix in tomatoes. Stir constantly.
- Mix in the broth along with the chicken and let everything cook approximately 4 minutes.
- Mix in remaining spices.
- Stir well. Let everything cook 2 additional minutes
- Mix in the chopped cilantro.
- Boil and turn the burner to low.
- Mix in cream cheese until it melts in.
- Boil for another 5 minutes.
- Put into serving bowls and garnish with diced tomatoes and cilantro leaves.

Creamy Pumpkin Curry

Calories: 230 | Fat: 23g | Protein: 12g | Carbs: 7.2g | Fiber: 3g

This recipe needs 1 hour and 45 minutes to prepare and will make several servings.

What to Use

- Ginger (.25 inch chopped)
- Sugar pumpkin (1 small, halved, seeded)
- Turmeric powder (.5 T)
- Shrimp (2 pounds)
- Coconut milk (one, 14-ounce can refrigerated ahead of time for one day)
- Chicken stock (1 cup)
- Coconut oil (2 tablespoons)
- Carrots (2, chopped)
- Coriander (.5 tsp)
- Zucchinis (4 small, chopped)
- Yellow onion (1 medium, chopped)
- Salt (as desired)
- Pepper (as desired)
- Crushed garlic (1 tsp)

What to Do

- Ensure your oven is heated to 350 degrees Fahrenheit.
- In a baking dish, add in 1 c water and place the pumpkin halves face up.
- Bake for 60 minutes.
- Add the coconut oil to a large soup pot before placing it on top of a burner set to a medium heat and cook the carrots and onion until the onion is clear.
- Remove the cream from the coconut milk and place it into the pot with the onions and carrots. The cream raised to the top of the can when you refrigerated it. If you are using a protein such as chicken instead of shrimp, now is the time to add the chicken so as to give it more cooking time (and not overcook the zucchini later).
- Allow the cream melt and to mix with the onions and the carrots.
- Turn down the heat. Simmer.
- Meanwhile, scoop out the roasted pumpkin. Put it into a blender or food processor. Add in the remaining liquids and process thoroughly.

- Add the zucchini and the pumpkin mixture to the soup pot. Stir. Continue to simmer.
- Peel and devein the shrimp and add it to the soup. Cook for approximately 6 minutes until the shrimp are firm.
- Ladle into serving bowls. Top with fresh cilantro.

Eggplant Parmesan Boats

Calories:442 | Fat: 29g | Protein: 20g | Carbs: 24g | Fiber: 9g

The recipe needs 30 minutes of preparation time, 31 minutes of cooking time and serves 4.

What to Use

- Marinara sauce (1.5 c)
- Eggplants (two 6-inch long, cut in half lengthwise)
- Olive oil (.5 teaspoon)
- Italian sausage (.5 pound, casings removed)
- Onion (1 small, diced)
- Garlic (2 cloves, chopped)
- Salt (as desired)
- Pepper (as desired)
- Parmesan (.25 cup, grated)
- Basil (for garnish)
- Shredded mozzarella cheese (1 c)

What to Do

- Ensure your oven is heated to 400 degrees F.

- Remove the middle of the eggplant halves, leaving .5 inch around the sides. Chop the scooped-out part, and set the chopped part aside.
- Brush olive oil on the middle of the shells.
- Roast the shells in the oven, inside up, between 10 and 15 minutes. Set aside.
- Meanwhile, dice up the onion and put it in a sauce pan. Break up the sausage into the same sauce pan. Cook the sausage and onion about 10 minutes.
- Chop the garlic and add it to the sausage and onion, cooking 1 minute.
- Add the chopped eggplant to the sausage, onion, and garlic, cooking about 7 minutes or until tender.
- Add 1 cup of the marinara sauce and season as desired. Warm the sauce for 4 minutes. Remove from heat.
- Spread the other cup of marinara sauce on the insides of the eggplant shells.
- Fill the shells with the sausage sauce.
- Top off with the cheeses.
- Bake between 10 and 15 minutes or until the cheese has melted.
- Garnish with fresh basil.

Enchilada Chicken Mango Salad

Calories: 100 | Fat: 17g | Protein: 18g | Carbs: 7.6g | Fiber: 8g

This recipe needs 5 minutes to prepare and will make 1 serving.

What to Use

- Hearts of romaine (1 small head)
- Enchilada chicken (1 – 2 cups, cold)
- Mango (1, peeled and diced)
- Avocado (.5 avocado, diced)
- Salt and pepper (sprinkle)

What to Do

- Chop the romaine lettuce and put it onto a serving plate.
- Put the chicken on top of the lettuce.
- Put the mango and the avocado on top of the chicken.

Greek Salad (HoriatikiSalata)

Calories: 216 | Fat: 14.3g | Protein: 15g | Carbs: 13g | Fiber: 8g

This recipe needs 10 minutes to prepare and will make 2 servings.

What to Use

- Olive oil (2 T)
- Tomatoes (2 large, ripe, sliced)
- Cucumber (1 medium, chopped)
- Green pepper (1 sliced thin)
- Kalamata olives (16, pits removed)
- Feta cheese (8 ounces, sliced or crumbled)
- Onion (1 sliced thin)
- Oregano (1 teaspoon)

What to Do

- Slice up the tomatoes, cucumber, onion, green pepper, and feta cheese. Take the pit out of the olives.
- Mix all ingredients in a bowl except for the feta cheese and the oregano.

- Put salad on a plate. Top with the feta cheese. Drizzle with olive oil.

Grilled Chicken Wings, Greens and Salsa

Calories: 279 | Fat: 14.3g | Protein: 20g | Carbs: 13g | Fiber: 8g

This recipe needs 5 minutes to prepare, 40 minutes to cook, and will make several servings.

What to Use

- Chicken wings (3 pounds, separated)
- Greens (optional, as a side)
- Salsa (as needed)
- Chicken spice mix (enough to coat chicken)

What to Do

- Season the chicken with the spice.
- Bake the chicken at 375 degrees Fahrenheit for about 40 minutes.
- Serve with the greens and salsa.

Kale Stuffed Portobello Mushrooms

Calories: 318 | Fat: 22g | Protein: 21g | Carbs: 11g | Fiber: 12g

This recipe needs 2 minutes to prepare, 13 minutes to cook, and will make 1 - 2 servings.

What to Use

- Portobello mushrooms (8 large)
- Kale (6 ounces, fresh)
- Cheese (8 slices, your choice)
- Extra virgin olive oil (2 tablespoons)

What to Do

- Ensure your oven is heated to 375 degrees F.
- Add the mushrooms to a baking sheet with the bottom side up.
- Cover mushrooms in olive oil and coat well.
- Place the baking sheet in the oven and let the mushrooms cook 10 minutes.
- Take the mushrooms out of the oven.
- Add kale and a slice of cheese to each mushroom.

- Bake (or broil) another until the cheese is thoroughly melted. You could also add sun dried tomatoes and feta cheese when you add the kale.

Low-Carb Mu Shu Lettuce Wraps

Calories: 73 | Fat: 1g | Protein: 9g | Carbs: 8g | Fiber: 1g

This recipe needs 12 minutes of preparation time, 12 minutes of cooking time, and will make 14 servings.

What to Use (to Make the Wraps)
- Cooking spray (as needed)
- Ground turkey breast (1 pound, 99% fat-free)
- Hoisin sauce (.5 cup plus 2 tablespoons
- Ginger (1 tablespoon), or fresh-grated ginger root
- Unsweetened apple juice (.5 cup)
- Cabbage (5 cups)
- Carrots (1.5 cups, shredded)
- Boston lettuce (14 leaves, separated, washed, dried)

What to Use (to Make the Topping)
- Scallions (.5 cup, chopped)
- Asian plum sauce (.5 cup, optional)

What to Do
- Using cooking spray, coat a non-stick frying pan thoroughly.

- Add in the turkey and place the pan onto a burner turned to a high-medium heat and let it cook until it reaches an internal temperature of 165 degrees F.
- Add in apple juice, hoisin sauce, ginger, carrots, and cabbage. Cook about 5 minutes, constantly stirring, until the cabbage is crisp-tender.
- Putt .33 cup of turkey filling onto each lettuce leaf.
- Add scallions on top.
- Drizzle 1 teaspoon of plum sauce over each plate of food.

Nacho Salad

Calories: 180 | Fat: 15g | Protein: 12g | Carbs: 8g | Fiber: 6.8g

This recipe needs 30 minutes to prepare (if meat used is not already cooked), 3 minutes to broil and will make 1 serving.

What to Use (AND How to Layer the Salad for Broiling)

Bottom:
- Iceberg lettuce (2 cups, shredded), or cabbage slaw (shredded)

Cooked Meat over Lettuce:
- Ham (.6 c, hashed)
- Hamburger (.6 c, spicy), or pepperoni, chicken, Italian sausage, linguica, or andouille
- Corned beef (.6 c hashed)

Cheese over Meat:
- Mozzarella cheese (.25 cup)
- Cheddar cheese (.25 cup, shredded), or bleu cheese, feta cheese, or sharp cheddar cheese

<u>Veggies over Cheese:</u>

- Tomatoes (.5 cup, chopped)
- Yellow onion (.25 cup, chopped)
- Jalapeno (8 slices)
- Black olives (8 olives, sliced), or green olives, green onions, banana peppers, or tasted garlic

What to Do

- Cook/bake the various meat.
- Layer as listed above.
- Broil on high for 3 minutes, often checking to make sure the cheese does not burn.
- After the dish is broiled, top with the following items:

What to Use

- Salsa (.25 cup, fresh, optional)
- Guacamole (.25 cup, fresh, optional)
- Sour cream (.25 cup, full-fat, optional)

No-Potato Salad

Calories: 175 | Fat: 20g | Protein: 13.4g | Carbs: 4.4g | Fiber: 5.4g

This recipe needs 25 minutes to prepare and will make 15 servings.

What to Use

- Cauliflower (2 heads florets)
- Eggs (1 dozen, hard-boiled, diced)
- Brown mustard (1 tsp)
- Salt (as desired)
- Pepper (as desired)
- Red onion (.5 medium onion, finely diced)
- Celery stalks (6, sliced fine)
- Dill pickles (6, chopped)
- Mayonnaise (.5 c)
- Dried dill (2 tablespoons)
- Crushed garlic (1 tsp)

What to Do

- Fill the pressure cooker with 4 inches of water, put the cauliflower in the cooker, lock the lid. Cook for 2.5

minutes. Alternately, you may steam the cauliflower 8 minutes or until tender and not yet mushy.

- Remove from heat. Ensure pressure has dropped before removing the lid.
- Strain and rise the cauliflower before patting it dry.
- Break the florets into chunks and place the chunks in a large mixing bowl before adding in the crushed garlic, dried dill, mayonnaise, dill pickles, celery stalks, red onion, brown mustard and eggs. Season as desired.
- Chill a couple hours.

Shrimp and Avocado Salad

Calories: 180 | Fat: 14g | Protein: 16.3g | Carbs: 8.4g | Fiber: 6.4g

This recipe needs 10 minutes to prepare, 2 hours to marinade and will make 2-4   servings.

What to Use to Make the Salad
- Cilantro dressing
- Shrimp (1 pound, cooked, deveined, tail removed)
- Avocados (2 ripe)
- Lettuce (4 cups)

What to Do to Make the Salad
- Make the marinade (See below)
- Cover and marinate the shrimp in the refrigerator about 2 hours.
- Wash and dry the lettuce.
- Slice up the avocados and place on top of the lettuce.
- Put the shrimp on top.
- Pour the remaining marinade on top.

*What to Use (to Make the **Cilantro Dressing/Marinade**)*

- Lime juice (2 T)
- Coconut oil (2 T)
- Fresh cilantro (.5 c torn)
- Salt (as desired)
- Pepper (as desired)

*What to Do (to Make the **Cilantro Dressing/Marinade**)*

- Mix together in a bowl.

Shrimp Ceviche Stuffed Avocado

Calories: 254 | Fat: 16g | Protein: 18g | Fiber: 6g | Carbs: 13g

This recipe needs 2 hours and 30 minutes to prepare and will make 4 servings.

What to Use

- Shrimp (28 extra-large, cleaned, deveined)
- Red onion (.5 onion, sliced)
- Garlic (2 cloves, crushed)
- White vinegar (.3 c)
- Cherry tomatoes (12, halved)
- Cilantro (2 tablespoons, finely chopped)
- Kosher salt (1 teaspoon)
- Jalapeno (.5 pepper, finely diced)
- Clam juice (2 tablespoons)
- Cumin (.125 teaspoon)
- Black pepper (.125 teaspoon)
- Olive oil (1 T)
- Honey (.5 teaspoon)
- Arugula (4 cups)
- Avocados (2 medium)

What to Do

- Boil water before tossing in the shrimp. Let them cook until they turn opaque.
- Take the shrimp out of the boiling water and put them into ice water to stop further cooking.
- Separately, combine the clam juice, olive oil, honey, jalapeno, tomatoes, onions, garlic, cilantro, cumin vinegar in a mixing bowl and season as needed.
- Mix in the shrimp and coat well before letting the results chill for a minimum of 2 hours.
- When ready to serve prepare the avocados before cutting them in half.
- Split the arugula into the 4 dishes.
- Put half an avocado into each dish.
- Fill each avocado with .5 cup of the ceviche.
- Top each avocado with 7 pieces of shrimp.

Skinny Cheeseburger Salad

Calories: 242 | Fat: 9g | Protein: 25g | Fiber: 5g | Carbs: 20g

This recipe requires 9 minutes of preparation, 10 minutes of cooking time, and serves 6.

*What to Use (to Make the **Burger Crumble**)*
- Ground beef (1 pound, extra lean)
- Yellow onion (1 cup, diced)
- Worcestershire sauce (3 tablespoons)
- Lawry's seasoning salt (.5 teaspoon)
- Black pepper (to taste, fresh-ground)

*What to Use (to Make the **Salad**)*
- Romaine lettuce (24 cups)
- Cheddar cheese (.75 cup, reduced fat), or full-fat cheddar
- Tomatoes (3 cups, chopped)

What to Do

- Add the beef to a skillet before placing the skillet on a burner set to a high-medium heat and cook until browned.
- Remove the fat from the skillet.
- Put the meat back into the skillet. Add the Worcestershire sauce and the seasonings.
- Turn the burner down to a low heat. Let everything cook 5 minutes stirring regularly.
- To make one salad, line a salad plate with 4 cups of lettuce.
- Spoon .5 cup of the hamburger crumble on top.
- Drain the tomatoes. Put .5 cup of the drained tomatoes on the hamburger.
- Put 2 tablespoons of Thousand Island dressing over the tomatoes.
- Put 2 tablespoons of cheddar cheese on the top.

Thai Beef Salad

Calories: 291 | Fat: 13g | Protein: 28g | Carbs: 18g | Fiber: 3g

This recipe requires 15 minutes preparation, 14 minutes of cooking time, and will serve 4.

What to Use

- Lime juice (.3 c)
- Sugar (2 T) or sugar substitute
- Mint (.25 cup, fresh, chopped and divided)
- Flank steak (1 pound, trimmed)
- Red bell pepper (1 cup, cut into strips)
- Carrot (.5 cup, shredded)
- Fish sauce (2 T)
- Cucumber (.5 small, peeled, sliced thin)
- Jalapeno pepper (.5 pepper, minced)
- Dry-roasted peanuts (.25 cup, unsalted, coarsely chopped)
- Watercress (4 cups, trimmed), or arugula
- Onion (5. C sliced thin)

What to Do

- Combine the fish sauce, sugar, half of the mint and lime juice together in a small mixing bowl.
- Put steaks on whatever you will broil it in.
- Spoon 2 tablespoons of this dressing over the steak. Turn the steak over to coat the other side.
- Broil the steak 7 minutes. Turn the steak over and broil it 7 more minutes or until cooked through (depends on thickness).
- Meanwhile, combine the salad ingredients of onion, carrot, cucumber, jalapeno, red bell pepper, and the remaining fresh mint. Put the salad onto the serving plates. Add the watercress on each plate.
- When the steak is fully cooked, remove it from the oven and let it cool approximately 4 minutes. Then cut the steak diagonally into very thin slices.
- Top the salad with the steak prior to serving.
- Top with the peanuts.

Tuna-Stuffed Tomatoes

Calories: 169 | Fat: 10g | Protein: 13g | Carbs: 8g | Fiber: 2g

This recipe needs 15 minutes to prepare and will make 4 servings.

What to Use

- Tomatoes (8 small)
- Tuna (two 3-ounce cans, oil-packed, drained)
- Kalamata olives (10 pitted, minced)
- Capers (1 T, drained, rinsed)
- Coconut oil (1 T)
- Thyme leaves (.5 teaspoon, fresh, minced)
- Fresh parsley (2 T minced)
- Salt (as desired)
- Pepper (as desired)

What to Do

- Put paper towels on a baking sheet.
- Remove the tops from the tomatoes. Remove the insides while leaving the tomato whole. Put the tomatoes upside down on the paper towels to drain.

- Combine tuna, capers, coconut oil and thyme in a bowl and mix well. Season as needed.
- Stuff each tomato with the tuna mixture.

Veggie Lasagna Stuffed Portobello Mushrooms

Calories: 236 | Fat: 13g | Protein: 20g | Carbs: 13g | Fiber: 1.8g

This recipe needs 28 minutes of preparation, 20 minutes cooking time, and will serve 4.

What to Use

- Olive oil (1 teaspoon)
- Baby spinach (2 cups, chopped)
- Garlic (3 cloves, chopped)
- Onion (.33 cup, chopped)
- Red bell pepper (.33 cup, chopped)
- Kosher salt (to taste)
- Ricotta (.75 cup, part skim)
- Parmesan cheese (.5 cup, grated)
- Egg (1 large)
- Basil leaves (4 large, chopped)
- Portobello mushroom caps (4 large)
- Marinara sauce (.5 cup)
- Mozzarella (.5 cup, part skim, shredded)

- Ensure your oven is heated to 400 degrees F.
- Coat a baking sheet with cooking spray.
- Take the stems off of the mushrooms.
- Scoop out the gills of the mushrooms.
- Spray the tops of the mushrooms with oil.
- Season as desired.
- Add the oil to the skillet before placing it on top of a burner set to a high-medium heat.
- Chop red pepper, garlic, onion and the baby spinach.
- Add the onion, garlic, and the red pepper to the skillet and let it cook 3 or 4 minutes or until soft.
- Season with .125 teaspoon salt.
- Add the baby spinach and sauté about 1 minute until wilted.
- Combine the egg, parmesan and ricotta cheese in a mixing bowl and season as desired.
- Stuff mushrooms with the results.
- Top with marinara sauce and 2 tablespoons of mozzarella.
- Bake between 20 and 25 minutes.
- Garnish with basil.

Chapter 4: Dinner Recipes

Burger hold the bun

Calories: 320 | Fat: 24g | Protein: 22g | Carbs: 3.1g | Fiber: 4g

This recipe requires 6 minutes of preparation, 12 minutes of cooking time, and will make 1 serving.

What to Use
- Butter (1 tablespoon)
- Hamburger (1 patty)
- Cheddar cheese (enough to cover patty)
- Cream cheese (enough to cover patty)
- Salsa (to taste, optional)
- Spices (to taste)
- Spinach (a few leaves)
- Salt (as desired)
- Pepper (as desired)

What to Do

- Add the butter to the skillet before placing the skillet on a burner turned to a medium heat.
- Add burger and season as needed. Cook both sides of the burger until it is almost cooked.
- Add the cheeses on the top. Turn down the heat and wait for cheeses to melt.
- Put spinach on top of the melted cheese. Pour some pan juices on top of the spinach if desired.
- Top with salsa.

Carolina BBQ Meatballs

Calories: 92 | Fat: 7g | Protein: 6g | Carbs: 1g | Fiber: .4g

This recipe needs 30 minutes to prepare, 3 minutes to cook, and will make 16 meatballs (4 servings).

What to Use (for the Meatballs)

- Ground pork (1 pound)
- Sugar (1 teaspoon) or sugar substitute
- Paprika (As desired)
- Salt (as desired)
- Pepper (as desired)
- Cumin (.5 teaspoon)
- Celery salt (.25 teaspoon)
- Egg (1)
- Cayenne pepper (.25 teaspoon)
- Almond flour (.25 cup)
- Water (1 tablespoon)

What to Use (for the BBQ Sauce)

- Yellow mustard (.25 cup)
- Frank's Hot Sauce (2 teaspoons)

- Dried onion flakes (1 tablespoon)
- Sugar (3 tablespoons) or sugar substitute
- Apple cider vinegar (2 tablespoons)
- Low-sugar ketchup (2 tablespoons)
- Salt (as desired)
- Pepper (as desired)

What to Do

- In a saucepan, combine the ketchup, apple cider vinegar, sugar, dried onion flakes, Frank's hot sauce and mustard and mix thoroughly before seasoning as desired. Place the saucepan on a burner turned to a low heat and let the sauce simmer for about 8 minutes.
- Combine all meatball ingredients in a bowl. Mix thoroughly.
- Form into 16 meatballs.
- Add a few meatballs to the skillet before placing it over a burner set to a medium heat, cook them for 3-4 minutes per side.
- Using parchment paper, cover a baking sheet.

- Place the bowl of sauce nearby and cover each meatball before placing them on the baking sheet.
- Broil for 2 – 3 minutes.
- Serve with coleslaw.

Cheese Enchiladas

Calories: 376 | Fat: 32g | Protein: 25g | Carbs: 8g | Fiber: 2g

This recipe needs 30 minutes to prepare, 20 minutes to cook, and will make 12 enchiladas (six 2-enchilada servings).

What to Use (to Make the Shells)
- Cauliflower (3 cups from one 16-ounce bag, frozen and thawed, drained, diced)
- Eggs (3)
- Mozzarella cheese (3 cups), or Monterey Jack cheese

What to Use (to Make Enchilada Sauce)
- Onion (.5 cup, chopped)
- Garlic (2 large cloves, chopped and crushed)
- Chili powder (1 tablespoon)
- Oil (4 tablespoons, healthy oil)
- Oregano (1 teaspoon)
- Pizza sauce (1 cup)
- Cheddar cheese (2 cups, shredded)
- Pepper Jack (2 cups, shredded), or Monterey Jack
- Cumin (2 tsp)

- Salt (as desired)
- Pepper (as desired)

What to Do

- Preheat oven to 450 degrees Fahrenheit.
- Mix the cauliflower, cheese, and eggs.
- Put the mixture onto two cookie sheets in .33 cup amounts, making twelve 6-inch flat rounds.
- Bake each sheet for approximately 15 minutes or until the edges brown.
- Let cool. Then loosen them. Let set.
- Meanwhile, start making the sauce by chopping the onions and garlic cloves, and shredding the cheese.
- Add 4 T coconut oil to a skillet before placing it on top of a burner turned to a medium heat.
- Add in chili powder, garlic and onion, garlic and let every cook for approximately 5 minutes.
- Mix in the tomato sauce and season as desired. Stir just until heated.
- Mix the cheeses.
- Get out a 9x13" casserole dish.
- Dredge each shell through the sauce and lay into the casserole dish golden side up.

- Put .25 cup of the mixed cheddar and jack cheeses or of Monterrey Jack cheese into each shell.
- Roll each shell and place them into the pan facing downward.
- Add the rest of the sauce and cheese to the top.
- Place the dish into the oven and let it bake for 20 minutes.
- As an option, you can top the baked enchiladas with shredded lettuce, chopped fresh tomatoes, and olives.

Cheesy Tuna Casserole

Calories: 459 | Fat: 33g | Protein: 31g | Carbs: 12g | Fiber: 4g

This recipe requires 20 minutes of preparation time, will cook in 5 minutes, and will serve 4.

What to Use

- Tuna (two 6-ounce cans, drained)
- Green beans (16-ounce bag, French-cut, frozen)
- Mushrooms (3 ounces, fresh, sliced)
- Butter (2 tablespoons)
- Chicken broth (.5 cup)
- Heavy cream (.75 cup)
- Onion (2 T chopped fine)
- Salt and pepper (to taste)
- Xanthan gum (optional)
- Celery (1 stalk, hashed fine)
- Cheddar cheese (4-8 ounces, shredded)

What to Do

- Cook the green beans in a medium pot. Drain well.

- Place the butter, celery, mushrooms and onion in a
  pan and place the pan on top of the stove over a
  burner turned to a medium heat and let everything
  cook for 5 minutes.
- Add the broth. Boil, letting the liquid cook down by
  half.
- Stir in the cream. Let come back up to a boil.
- Turn down the heat until the sauce is thickened,
  stirring frequently. Don't let it boil over.
- Season to taste.
- Put the mushroom and tuna mixture into the green
  beans.
- Add salt and pepper if needed.
- Put the cheese in it, thoroughly mixing it in.
- Put the mixture into a 1.5 or 2-quart casserole dish.
- Microwave or bake until hot.

Chicken Cacciatore with Spaghetti Squash

Calories: 267 | Fat: 5.1g | Protein: 40g | Carbs: 17g | Fiber: 3.6g

This recipe needs 1.5 hours to prepare and will make 6 servings.

What to Use

- Chicken thighs (4 boneless, skinless, bite-size)
- Onion (1 medium, diced)
- Bell peppers (1 large, bite-size)
- Garlic (2 cloves, minced)
- Dried thyme (.5 tsp)
- Chicken stock (1 cup)
- Diced tomatoes (one 28-ounce can)
- Tomato sauce (one 8-ounce can)
- Dried basil (.5 tsp.)
- Salt (as desired)
- Pepper (as desired)
- Yellow squash (.5, diced)
- Dried oregano (.5 tsp)
- Spaghetti squash (1, small)

What to Do

- Dice the veggies. Set them aside.
- Cut the chicken up. Season it as desired.
- Place the chicken in a Dutch oven and let it brown for about 8 minutes.
- Add in the onion, garlic and bell pepper and let them cook for approximately 5 minutes or until the onions soften.
- Add the chicken tomato sauce, tomatoes, and the chicken stock.
- Season as desired and mix well before letting everything boil.
- Turn the heat to low and let everything cook for 30 minutes.
- Add the yellow squash. Cook between 15 and 30 more minutes.

Chicken Curry

Calories: 997 | Fat: 52g | Protein: 86g | Carbs: 17g | Fiber: 4g

This recipe needs 30 minutes to prepare, 40 minutes to cook, and will make 1 servings.

What to Use

- Chicken breasts (1.5 breasts)
- Cauliflower (1 head)
- Onion powder (.5 tsp.)
- Thai Kitchen Lite Coconut Milk (1 can)
- Hot curry powder (2 tablespoons)
- Garam masala (1 tablespoon)
- Ghee (.5 tablespoon)
- Green beans (2 c, frozen)
- Garlic powder (.5 tsp)
- Salt (as desired)
- Pepper (as desired)

What to Do

- Cut up the chicken into chunks.

- Coat the chicken chunks in half curry powder and half garam masala.
- Sear chicken in butter in frying pan.
- Take the chicken out of the pan and put it into a deep pot. Leave the burned pieces and butter in the frying pan because they are flavorful.
- Add coconut milk to the frying pan and scratch off all of the burned bits.
- Pour the coconut milk and the burned bits over the chicken that is in the deep pot.
- Add the remaining spices.
- Boil on a low-medium heat for half an hour.
- Add green beans. Continue cooking, uncovered to let the sauce thicken.
- Meanwhile, boil the cauliflower in water and 1 tablespoon of butter in a separate pot.
- Mash the cauliflower until it is in small pieces. Season as needed.

Crispy Carnitas (Succulent, Caramelized Pork)

Calories: 280 | Fat: 32g | Protein: 15g | Carbs: 4.2g | Fiber: 8g

This recipe needs 20 minutes to prepare, 3 – 4 hours to cook, and will make 6   servings.

What to Use

- Chili powder (1 tsp)
- Boneless pork shoulder or butt (3 – 4 pounds, cut into 5 pieces)
- Salt (as desired)
- Pepper (as desired)
- Cinnamon stick (.5)
- Bay leaf (2)
- Garlic (4 cloves, thinly sliced)
- Onion (1, chopped)
- Water (enough to braise with)
- Cumin (1 tsp)

What to Do

- Preheat oven to 350 degrees Fahrenheit.

- Mix the cumin, chili powder, and the salt together in a bowl. Rub this mixture all over the meat.
- Put the meat into a large oven proof pot. Note: The braising step could be done in a slow cooker.
- Almost cover the meat in water.
- Add the garlic, onion, cinnamon stick and the bay leaf.
- Braise for 3 – 3.5 hours in the oven, uncovered and stirring the meat a few times. The meat will be done when it is tender, slightly browned, and most of the liquid is gone.
- Take the pot out of the oven.
- Cut the meat on a cutting board or shred it by hand into strips.
- Take the cinnamon stick and the bay leaf out of the pot.
- Put the shredded meat back into the pot (or onto a roasting pan or baking sheet) with its juices. Put the meat back into the oven.
- Roast the meat until it is dark and crispy. Alternatively, you could broil it to speed things up.
- Note: The meat could be cooked ahead of time and the crisping step done just before serving.

Crispy Fried Salmon

Calories: 337 | Fat: 19.5g | Protein: 29.7g | Carbs: 8g | Fiber: 19.5g

This recipe can be prepared in 4 minutes, will cook in 30 minutes, and will serve 4.

What to Use

- Chicken broth (850 milliliters, lightly seasoned)
- Fennel (7 bulbs)
- Coconut oil (2 T)
- Salmon Steak (4 x 120 g)
- Salt (as desired)
- Pepper (as desired)
- Broad beans (90 g)
- Basil (1 handful)
- Peas (100 g, podded)
- Mint (2 small handfuls)
- Green beans (100 g)

What to Do

- Make the aioli (See recipe below). Set aside.

- Add the stock to a large pot before placing the pot on the stove over a burner turned to high heat.
- Mix in the fennel and boil 4 more minutes.
- Meanwhile, heat up a non-stick frying pan.
- Using olive oil, pat the steak and season as needed. Put them in the pan with the skin facing downward. Let them cook for 5 minutes, flip and cook an additional minute. They will change color when they are cooked.
- Once the fennel is cooked, add in the beans and cook an additional 2 minutes.
- Turn the salmon steaks back over for their last minute of cooking. Remove from fire. Don't overcook the fish.
- Back to the fennel mixture, add the peas and other veggies. Cook for 2 more minutes.
- Plate the vegetables in fourths, top using the basil as well as the mint and top it all with the steak. Top with aioli prior to serving.

*What to Use (for **Aioli** Topping for the Fried Salmon)*
- Garlic (.5 small clove, peeled)
- Salt (as desired)
- Pepper (as desired)

- Coconut oil (285 milliliters)
- Olive oil (285 milliliters)
- Lemon juice (to taste)
- Spicy mustard (1 tsp)

*What to Do (to Make the **Aioli** Topping for the Fried Salmon)*

- Mash the garlic. Mix with 1 teaspoon salt.
- In a small mixing bowl, whisk together egg yolk and mustard before adding in both oils.
- Add the lemon juice after the mixture thickens before seasoning as needed. Add more lemon juice if desired.
- Good with fish (a classic with salmon), chicken, pork, salad and in seafood soups.

Greek Style Salmon with Avocado Tzatziki

Calories: 373 | Fat: 22.2g | Protein: 36g | Carbs: 10.5g | Fiber: 4g

This recipe can be prepared in 25 minutes, can be cooked in 10 minutes, and serves 4.

What to Use

- Salmon (24 ounces, cut into 4 pieces)
- Lemon zest (2 teaspoons)
- Yogurt (2 tablespoons)
- Garlic (.5 cloves, grated)
- Oregano (1 teaspoon)
- Salt (.25 teaspoon)
- Pepper (.25 teaspoon)
- Avocado tzatziki (2 cups)
- Coconut oil (2 T)
- Lemon juice (1.5 T)

What to Do

- Mix together the oil, lemon juice, lemon zest, yogurt, oregano, garlic, salt, and pepper.

- Marinate the fish in the mixture for 1 hour.
- Ensure your oven is set to 400 degrees F.
- Prepare a glass baking dish and then add in the fish.
- Bake about 10 minutes (when fish starts to flake easily).
- Top with avocado tzatziki.

Ground Beef and Bell Peppers

Calories: 380 | Fat: 22g | Protein: 25g | Carbs: 6.2g | Fiber: 4g

This recipe can be prepared in 11 minutes, cooked in 12, and will serve 2.

What to Use

- Onion (1, diced)
- Coconut oil (enough to fry with)
- Ground beef (1 pound)
- Spinach (1 cup, fresh, chopped)
- Salt and pepper or a spice mix (to taste), or chili powder and black pepper if you want it spicy
- Bell pepper (1 red, sliced)

What to Do

- Chop the spinach. Set aside.
- Dice the onion into tiny pieces.
- Add the oil to a skillet before placing the skillet on the stove over a burner set to a medium heat. Add in the onion and coat well in oil. Let it cook for 60 seconds.

- Mix in the spinach and the beef and stir well. Season as desired.
- Stir fry everything until cooked.
- Put the sliced fresh bell pepper on a serving plate, and dish up the cooked meat mixture beside the peppers.

Hamburger Patties with Creamy Tomato Sauce, Fried Cabbage

Calories: 320 | Fat: 26g | Protein: 22g | Carbs: 5.1g | Fiber: 8g

This recipe requires 15 minutes of preparation, will cook in 20 minutes, and serves 4.

What to Use (to Make the Hamburger Patties)
- Ground beef (1.5 pounds)
- Egg (1)
- Feta cheese (3.25 ounces)
- Salt (as desired)
- Pepper (as desired)
- Parsley (.75 ounces, fresh, finely chopped)
- Olive oil (1 tablespoon)
- Butter (1 ounce)

What to Use (to Make the Gravy)
- Heavy whipping cream (1.25 cups)
- Parsley (1.75 ounces, fresh, coarsely chopped)
- Tomato paste (2 tablespoons)
- Pepper (as desired)

- Salt (as desired)

Fried Green Cabbage

- Green cabbage (1.5 pounds, shredded)
- Butter (4.25 ounces)
- Salt and pepper

What to Do

- Make the cabbage first: Sauté the shredded cabbage in melted butter for at least 15 minutes.
- Combine hamburger ingredients together in a mixing bowl. Form 8 oblong patties.
- Add the olive oil and butter to a skillet before placing the skillet on the stove over a burner turned to a high-medium heat.
- Fry the hamburger patties for at least 10 minutes.
- When the patties are almost cooked through, pour the whipping cream and the tomato paste into the frying pan. Stir and bring to a boil.
- Sprinkle parsley on top just before serving.

Meat-Based Pizza

Calories: 195 | Fat: 24g | Protein: 17g | Carbs: 1.2g | Fiber: .5g

This recipe needs 15 minutes to prepare, 40 minutes to cook, and will make 1   serving.

What to Use

- Ground beef (small package, uncooked)
- Salsa (to taste)
- Onion (.5 to 1 onion, diced)
- Spices (to taste, Italian or other)
- Garlic powder (to taste)
- Mozzarella cheese (to taste, shredded), or other cheese
- Bacon (4 – 6 strips)

What to Do

- Dice onion and put the onion into a baking dish.
- Add the beef, salsa, garlic powder and other spices into a baking dish. Mix together.
- Shred the cheese and put it evenly over the top of the beef mixture.

- Cut the bacon into small pieces and put the pieces on top of the cheese.
- Ensure your oven is set to 375 degrees F
- Place the pizza in the oven and let it cook for 35 minutes.

Mexican Casserole

Calories: 69 | Fat: 30g | Protein: 3.56g | Carbs: 4.5g | Fiber: .65g

This recipe can be prepared in 15 minutes, will cook in 30 minutes, and will make 12 servings.

What to Use

- Cumin (.5 tsp)
- Cauliflower (1 head)
- Onion (.5 white)
- Chili powder (.5 tsp)
- Green bell pepper (1 hashed)
- Parmesan (1.5 cups)
- Bell pepper (1 hashed)
- Cherry tomatoes (4, cut in half)

What to Do

- Ensure your oven is set to 350 degrees Fahrenheit.
- Place the skillet on top of the stove over a burner set to a medium heat.

- Roast the chili powder, pepper, cumin and onion, stirring regularly until the veggies are fully cooked.
- Dice the cauliflower. Cook it in the microwave for 3 minutes.
- Put the tomatoes and 1 cup of the cheese in with the cauliflower. Mix.
- Mix the results with the vegetables.
- Using cooking spray coat a baking dish.
- Add the vegetable mixture to the baking dish.
- Add the rest of the cheese.
- Place the dish in the oven and let it cook for approximately 40 minutes.
- Garnish as desired.

Moroccan Meatballs

Calories: 280 | Fat: 32g | Protein: 15g | Carbs: 4.2g | Fiber: 8g

This recipe can be prepared in 14 minutes, cooked in 60 minutes, and serves 7 (about 36 meatballs).

*What to Use (to Make the **Meatballs**)*

- Parsley (2 tablespoons, fresh, minced)
- Pepper (as desired)
- Salt (as desired)
- Cumin (1 tsp.)
- Lamb (1.75 pounds, ground)
- Paprika (.5 T)

*What to Do (To Make the **Meatballs**)*

- Mix together the paprika, cumin and parsley and season as needed.
- Crumble the ground lamb into the bowl.
- Wash your hands. Knead all ingredients together.
- Scoop meatballs with tablespoon and level off. Form round meatballs from the scooped meat and line them up on a baking sheet.

*What to Use (to Make the **Sauce**)*

- Paprika (1 tsp)
- Coconut oil (1 tablespoon)
- Onions (2 cups, diced)
- Garlic (2 teaspoons, fresh, minced)
- Pepper (as desired)
- Salt (as desired)
- Tomatoes (2 cups, diced)
- Water (1.5 cups)
- Tomato paste (.66 cup)
- Cumin (1 tsp ground)
- Parsley leaves (2 tablespoons, fresh, minced)
- Pistachios (.25 cup, roasted, chopped, for garnish)

*What to Do (to Make the **Sauce** and to Finish Making the Meatball Dish)*

- Heat up the oil in a deep fry pan.
- Sauté onion 5 minutes.
- Mix together garlic, cumin, paprika, salt, and pepper. Stir ingredients in.
- Mix in tomato paste. Stir about 1 minute.
- Add water, tomatoes, and parsley. Stir to mix.
- Boil the sauce.

- Place the meatballs in the pan.
- Cover the sauce. Turn the heat to low before letting everything cook approximately 45 minutes.
- Uncover and continue cooking 20 more minutes until the sauce is thickened.
- Dish up. Top with chopped pistachios.

No Bean Turkey and Sweet Potato Chili

Calories: 235 | Carbs: 14 g | Protein: 23 g | Fat: 8 g | Fiber: 2 g

This recipe needs 10 minutes to prepare, 40 minutes to cook, and will make 5 servings.

What to Use

- Ground turkey (20 ounces, lean, ground)
- Kosher salt (to taste)
- Onion (.5 cup, chopped)
- Garlic (3 cloves, crushed)
- Rotel mild tomatoes with green chilies (10-ounce can)
- Tomato sauce (8-ounce can)
- Water (.75 cup)
- Cumin (.5 teaspoon)
- Chili powder (.25 teaspoon)
- Paprika (.25 teaspoon)
- Bay leaf (1)
- Sweet potato (1 medium, peeled, diced into .5-inch cubes)
- Cilantro (as desired for garnish)

What to Do

- Put turkey, salt, and cumin in a large skillet and brown over medium-high heat. Crumble with a spatula into smaller pieces as it cooks. Completely cook through.
- Reduce the heat to medium. Add the onion and garlic and cook another 3 minutes.
- Add the can of Rotel tomatoes, the sweet potatoes, tomato sauce, water, paprika, chili powder, cumin, salt, and the bay leaf.
- Cover. Simmer over medium-low heat about 25 minutes or until the potatoes are soft.
- Add .25 cup of water (more if needed). Remove the bay leaf.

Parsley and Garlic Chicken with Broccoli

Calories: 486 | Carbs: 15.7 g | Protein: 54 g | Fat: 19 g | Fiber: - g

This recipe needs 30 minutes to prepare and will make 4 - 5 servings.

What to Use

- Chicken cutlets (8-10 pieces, organic)
- Whole wheat pastry flour (.33 cup)
- Olive oil (3 tablespoons)
- Dry white wine (.75 cup)
- Butter (2 tablespoons, cut into pieces)
- Garlic (4 cloves, chopped)
- Celtic salt (.25 teaspoon)
- Broccoli florets (16 ounces, fresh)

What to Do

- Put the flour into a shallow bowl or plate.
- Coat the chicken with the flour.
- Turn on the stove to medium-high. Heat up half of the olive oil in a large nonstick skillet.
- Cook the chicken about 4 minutes per side.

- Meanwhile, microwave the broccoli for about 6 minutes.
- Take the chicken out of the pan and put onto a serving plate.
- Add the garlic to the skillet. Cook for 30 seconds to 1 minute.
- Add wine to the skillet. Cook about 3 minutes until the liquid is reduced by half.
- Turn off the heat.
- Add the butter, parsley and the salt.
- Pour this mixture over the chicken.

Pesto Chicken Casserole with Feta Cheese

Calories: - | Carbs: - g | Protein: - g | Fat: - g | Fiber: - g

This recipe needs 15 minutes to prepare, 30 minutes to cook, and will make 4 servings.

What to Use

- Chicken breasts (1.5 pounds, chopped)
- Pesto (3.5 ounces, red or green)
- Heavy whipping cream (1.66 cups)
- Olives (8 tablespoons, pitted)
- Garlic (1, finely chopped)
- Salt and pepper (to taste)
- Butter (enough to fry with)
- Leafy greens (.33 pound)
- Olive oil (to taste)
- Sea salt (to taste)

What to Do

- Preheat the oven to 400 degrees Fahrenheit.
- Cut the chicken into small pieces. Season.
- Fry the chicken until it is golden brown.
- In a bowl, mix the pesto and the heavy cream.

- Put the chicken pieces into a baking dish.
- Put the feta cheese, garlic, olive and the pesto-cream mixture in with the chicken.
- Bake between 20 and 30 minutes or until the food becomes a light brown around the edges.
- Serve with a side of romaine lettuce or else slightly sautéed asparagus or green beans, as possible suggestions.

Pizza Topping Casserole

Calories: 582 | Carbs: 5 g | Protein: 27 g | Fat: 50 g | Fiber: 1 g

This recipe needs 30 minutes to prepare, 2 hours to cook (including homemade sauce) and will make 6 - 8 servings.

What to Use

- Italian sausage (1 pound, bulk)
- Heavy cream (.5 cup)
- Garlic powder (.25 teaspoon)
- Green pepper (.5 cup, chopped)
- Red onion (.5 cup, slivered)
- Italian seasoning (.5 teaspoon) and/or basil
- Mozzarella cheese (8 ounces, whole milk, cubed)
- Pizza sauce (.25 cup, See recipe below)
- Pepperoni (3.5 ounces, chopped)
- Mushrooms (8 ounces, fresh)
- Red pepper (as desired, crushed, optional)
- Eggs (4)

What to Do

- Make the pizza sauce using the recipe below.

- Chop and sliver the veggies. Cube the cheese. Set aside.
- Brown the sausage and mushrooms. Drain off the grease.
- Whisk the eggs, cream, sauce, and the seasoning together in a bowl. Set aside.
- Grease a 7 x 9-inch deep baking pan.
- Put the Italian sausage, mushrooms, pepperoni, green pepper and the cheese into the baking pan.
- Pour the egg mixture over the meat mixture. Mix well.
- Top the meat mixture with the red onion.
- Sprinkle with Italian seasoning, garlic powder, and crushed red pepper.
- Bake at 350 degrees Fahrenheit between 45 and 55 minutes or until an inserted knife comes out almost clean.
- Let stand and cool 5 minutes before you dish it up.

*What to Use (to Make the **Pizza Sauce**)*
- Tomato sauce (8-ounce can)
- Tomato paste (2 tablespoons)
- Water (.5 cup)

- Splenda (2 teaspoons, granular), or equivalent liquid Splenda
- Garlic powder (.25 teaspoon)
- Dried basil (.5 teaspoon or to taste)

*What to Do (to Make the **Pizza Sauce**)*

- Put all ingredients together into a saucepan and bring to a boil.
- Partially cover pan. Reduce heat and simmer for 1 hour.
- Note: Makes one cup and can be frozen.

Pizza Sauce - *Calories: 22 | Carbs: 5 g | Protein: 1 g | Fat: 0 g | Fiber: 1 g*

Rosemary Oven-Fried Chicken

Calories: 248 | Carbs: 1.8 g | Protein: 27.4 g | Fat: 8.7 g | Fiber: 1.1 g

This recipe needs 15 minutes to prepare, 25 minutes to cook, and will make 4 servings.

What to Use

- Buttermilk (.25 cup, nonfat)
- Dijon mustard (2 tablespoons)
- Chicken (four 4-ounce)
- Whole wheat panko (.33 cup; these are Japanese breadcrumbs)
- Dry-roasted cashews (.33 cup, finely chopped)
- Rosemary (.75 teaspoon, fresh, minced)
- Kosher salt (.25 teaspoon)
- Black pepper (.25 teaspoon, freshly ground)
- Red pepper (.25 teaspoon, ground)
- Cooking spray (enough to coat)
- Honey (4 teaspoons)

What to Do

- Preheat oven to 425 degrees Fahrenheit.

- In a bowl, mix together the buttermilk and mustard.
- Add the chicken and coat all sides of the chicken.
- Heat a small skillet over medium-high heat.
- Add the panko to the skillet. Stirring frequently, cook 3 minutes until golden.
- Combine the panko, cashews, rosemary, kosher salt, black pepper, and red pepper in a shallow dish.
- Dredge the chicken in the panko mixture.
- Put the chicken in a foil-lined jelly-roll pan.
- Bake at 425 degrees for 25 minutes or until the chicken is done.
- Drizzle the chicken with honey.

Shrimp Scampi over Noodles

Calories: 170 | Carbs: 12 g | Protein: 11 g | Fat: 7 g | Fiber: 4 g

This recipe needs 15 minutes to prepare and will make 2 servings.

What to Use
- Zucchini (3 cups)
- Butter (2 tablespoons)
- Garlic (2 tablespoons, minced)
- Red pepper flakes (.125 crushed, optional)
- Shrimp (12 large, shelled, deveined)
- White wine (2.5 tablespoons), or reduced-sodium chicken broth
- Lemon juice (1.5 tablespoons)
- Parmesan cheese (2 tablespoons, grated)

What to Do

- Make the zucchini noodles with a julienne peeler, vegetable spiral, or mandolin.
- Heat up the butter over medium-low heat. Add the red pepper and the garlic. Cook just 1 minute, stirring constantly.
- Add the shrimp to the pan. Cook about 2 minutes or until they are cooked through.
- Season.
- Turn up the heat to medium.
- Add lemon juice and white wine. While heating up, scrape brown bits from pan bottom.
- Add the shrimp and the zucchini noodles. Stir about 30 seconds.
- Divide the noodles among 2 plates. Put 6 shrimp on each plate, and sprinkle with 1 teaspoon of Parmesan on each plate of shrimp.

Simple Herb Crusted Salmon

Calories: - | Carbs: - g | Protein: - g | Fat: - g | Fiber: - g

This recipe needs 20 minutes to prepare, 15 minutes to cook, and will make 2   servings.

What to Use (to Make the Salmon)

- Salmon (2 6-ounce fillets)
- Coconut flour (1 tablespoon)
- Parsley (2 tablespoons, fresh or dried)
- Olive oil (1 tablespoon)
- Dijon mustard (1 tablespoon)
- Salt and pepper (to taste)

What to Use (to Make the Salad)

- *Arugula (2 cups)*
- *Red onion (.25 onion, thinly sliced)*
- *Lemon juice (juice of 1 lemon)*
- *White wine vinegar (1 tablespoon)*
- *Olive oil (1 tablespoon)*
- *Salt and pepper (to taste)*

What to Do

- Preheat the oven to 450 degrees Fahrenheit.
- Put foil or parchment on baking sheet.
- Put fillets on baking sheet.
- Put olive oil and Dijon mustard onto fillets. Rub into the fish.
- Mix together in a bowl, the salt, pepper, parsley, and the coconut flour.
- Sprinkle the flour mixture onto the salmon. Then hand pat into the fish.
- Bake between 10 and 15 minutes.
- Meanwhile, mix the salad ingredients together and place the salad onto 2 serving plates.
- Put the fish onto the plates.

Tasty Fried Chicken Breast

Calories: - | Carbs: - g | Protein: - g | Fat: - g | Fiber: - g

This recipe needs 10 minutes to prepare, 15 minutes to cook, and will make 1   servings.

What to Use

- Chicken breast (1)
- Butter (enough to stir fry with)
- Salt and pepper (to taste)
- Curry powder (to taste)
- Garlic powder (to taste)
- Greens (.5 cup)

What to Do

- Cut chicken into small chunks.
- Heat up the butter in a frying pan.
- Put the chicken into the pan. Stir to coat chicken.
- Add spices to taste.
- Stir fry until the chicken browns and gets crunchy.
- Serve with greens on the side.

Chapter 5: Snack Recipes

Chocolate Cupcakes

Calories: 374 g | Carbs: 3 g | Protein: 7.8 g | Fat: 36.1 g | Fiber: - g

This recipe needs 7 minutes to prepare, 35 minutes to cook, and will make 12   servings.

What to Use

- Ketocal powder (12 grams)
- Carb-free, sugar-free sweetener (to taste)
- Almond flour (10 grams)
- Water (1 milliliter)
- Baking powder (1 gram)
- Butter (14 grams)
- Coconut (14 grams)
- Cocoa powder (2 grams)
- Eggs (18, whisked)

What to Do

- Preheat the oven to 350 degrees Fahrenheit.

- Whisk the eggs.
- Mix all ingredients together, adding the sweetener to taste.
- Pour batter into baking cups.
- Cook between 30 and 35 minutes.

Chocolate Muffins

Calories: - | Carbs: 4 g | Protein: 12 g | Fat: 14 g | Fiber: 10 g

This recipe needs 8 minutes to prepare, 15 minutes to cook, and will make 12   servings.

What to Use

- Apple cider vinegar (5 milliliters)
- Coconut oil (25 milliliters)
- Caramel syrup (50 milliliters)
- Cocoa powder (5 ounces)
- Golden flaxseed (25 ounces)
- Cinnamon (1 tablespoon)
- Baking powder (.5 teaspoon)
- Salt (.5 teaspoon)
- Slivered almonds (4.5 ounces)

What to Do

- Preheat oven to 350 degrees Fahrenheit.
- Mix all dry ingredients (except for the almonds) together in a bowl.
- Mix all wet ingredients together in a bowl.

- Combine the dry and wet ingredients together.
- Pour mixture into muffin liners.
- Sprinkle almond slivers on top of each muffin.
- Bake muffins for 15 minutes.

Chocolate Protein Pudding

Calories: - | Carbs: 19 g | Protein: 30 g | Fat: 12 g | Fiber: 8 g

This recipe needs 8 minutes to prepare, 30 minutes to chill, and will make 2   servings.

What to Use

- Chia seeds (3 tablespoons)
- Almond milk (1 cup, unsweetened)
- Chocolate protein powder or cocoa powder (1 scoop)
- Raspberries (.25 cup, fresh)
- Honey (1 teaspoon, optional)

What to Do

- Mix the almond milk and the chocolate protein powder together, stirring well.
- Add the Chia seeds. Mix and let sit for 5 minutes, stirring occasionally.
- Put into 2 serving cups. Chill in fridge 30 minutes.
- Serve with honey on top if desired. Top with raspberries or another type of berry on top, or top with peanuts or some other nut if desired.

Coconut Cream Macaroons

Calories: 78 | Carbs: - g | Protein: - g | Fat: - g | Fiber: - g

This recipe needs 15 minutes to prepare, 55 minutes to cook, and will make several servings.

What to Use
- Heavy cream (3 ounces)
- Cream cheese (9 ounces)
- Vanilla (1 teaspoon)
- Egg whites (4 or 5)
- Cream of tartar (.25 teaspoon)
- Erythritol (1 cup)
- Salt (.125 teaspoon)
- Dried coconut (18 ounces)
- Unsweetened white chocolate syrup (to taste)
- Semi-sweet chocolate chips (to taste)

What to Do
- Preheat oven to 325 degrees Fahrenheit.
- Separate the yolks from the eggs.

- Whisk the egg whites, vanilla, cream of tartar, and the salt together, occasionally sprinkling in the erythritol. Whisk until the mixture peaks.

- Add coconut to the egg white mixture. Mix and set bowl aside.

- In a separate bowl, mix together the chocolate syrup, cream cheese, and the heavy cream. Mix ingredients well.

- Add the ingredients from the other bowl and mix all ingredients together.

- Add the chocolate chips after everything else is mixed. Scoop mixture onto a cookie sheet. Bake in preheated oven for about 25 minutes. Turn the oven off and let the cookies remain in the oven another 30 minutes, so they will dry.

High-Protein Tiramisu

Calories: 147 | Carbs: 10.8 g | Protein: 25.2 g | Fat: 5 g | Fiber: - g

This recipe needs 15 minutes in total to prepare, 30 minutes to cook, and will make several servings.

What to Use for the Sponge Cake Base
- Egg whites (6)
- Dymatize Nutrition Elite egg protein (35 grams)
- Cream of tartar (.25 teaspoon)
- Coconut flour (15 grams)

What to Use for the (Faux) Mascarpone Layer
- Fat-free quark (250 grams)
- Vanilla-flavored whey protein (28 grams)

What Else to Use
- Espresso (60 milliliters)
- Raw cocoa powder (1 teaspoon)

What to Do to Create the Sponge Cake
- Separate the egg yolks from the egg whites.

- Whip the egg whites together with the cream of tartar until it stiffens and peaks.

- In a separate mixing bowl, mix the coconut flour and protein powder together. Fold in gently to mix together with the egg white and cream of tartar mixture.

- Pour the sponge cake batter into a baking paper-lined pan.

- Bake between 20 and 30 minutes until browned and almost hard.

- Poke holes into the sponge cake. Pour coffee on it.

What to Do to Assemble the Cake

- Use a cake pan that is half the size of the one used for baking the cake.

- Cut the sponge cake down the middle, making two equal halves.

- Cut the sponge cake down the middle of each half, making four equal pieces.

- In a bowl, mix the whey protein and the quark.

- Put the first cake layer in the pan and spread one-quarter of the quark mixture on top. Dust the top with cocoa powder.

- Repeat the layering of the cake, the quark mixture and the cocoa powder for the other layers.
- Refrigerate overnight.

Conclusion

Thank you again for downloading this cookbook. I hope it was informative and that it will be able to provide you with a good head start on your new recipe collection that you need to have and use so that you can hopefully prevent most of the epileptic seizures that you or your child would otherwise have to endure. Many healthy, mouthwatering dishes await you here.

You or your child will also lose some weight while on this diet, which most of us would not mind, because of the restriction of carbohydrates. Get ready to go to the Goodwill store to purchase clothes in several different sizes because, if you or your child are overweight, the weight will fall off while on this diet.

The next step is to decide which one of the three main types of ketogenic diet that you need to be on (or to put your child on). Are you or your child sedentary, too obese to exercise at all, or unable to exercise? You may want to start off with the strict standard ketogenic diet plan. Will you or your child be exercising? You will want to follow the targeted ketogenic diet so that you or your child will have a little bit of energy during exercise.

Do you think you or your child will have a hard time sticking to this diet? Opt for the cyclical ketogenic diet. This last diet is similar to what Dolly Parton used several years ago to lose a lot of weight. She binged on weekends and was good on week days, and it worked out wonderfully for her.

Finally, if you found this book useful in any way, a review on Amazon would be appreciated!